THE OTHER END OF THE NEEDLE

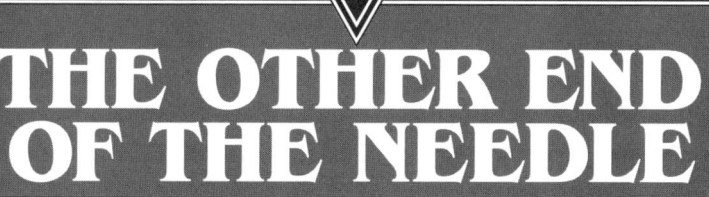

THE OTHER END OF THE NEEDLE

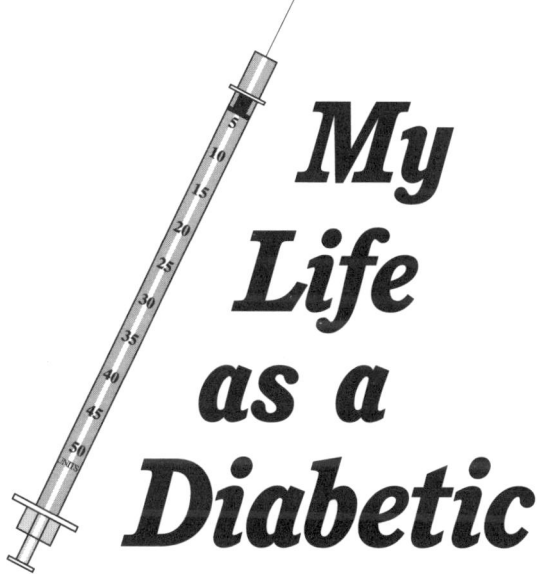

My Life as a Diabetic

By Mary Elizabeth Updike

Copyright © 1999
L. Wayne Updike
Independence, Missouri

Printed in the United States of America

For additional copies call
1-800-767-8181
1-816-373-4065

Contents

ACKNOWLEDGEMENTS

One of the common charac-
teristics found among people
who are dealing with health
problems is their natural desire
to tell others of their experiences, sometimes in great detail.
The brevity of this story,
when compared to the long
years it took to unfold, will attest
that I have successfully quelled
that tendency to a considerable
degree. Much more could have
been included about my life in
association with family, friends in
many places, and with some
wonderful people in the medical
profession.

But my purpose has not been simply to recount the personal history of my journey. Instead, I am hoping that my story will be of some help to others who may have a similarly difficult way to go in proceeding through this life.

My appreciation is deep for many who offered help, both spiritual and temporal, along the way. I know that my husband has provided help at a level without which I simply would not have survived so long. And of course the same may be said of many in the medical field.

The encouragement, and even urging, of Doctor William Quick, was significant in my getting started, and the major assistance of my husband in preparing the manuscript was a requirement for my completing it. He says he was compelled to get involved because his grandmother's name was Phoebe Dickens, and he was baptized by a minister named William Shakespeare.

If even one diabetic is assisted in arriving at a decision not to give up, but to just stay as optimistic as possible, and find the joy which comes from following through with such a decision, this minimal recounting of my experiences will have been worthwhile.

Mary Elizabeth Spike

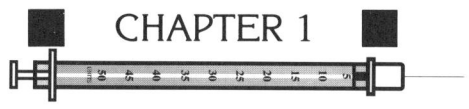

CHAPTER 1

THE FIRST ADJUSTMENT

"I refuse. I absolutely refuse. I will not be a diabetic." I stomped my foot and glared at Doctor Vance Link. He just smiled and reminded me that neither he nor I had any influence over that decision.

"Your blood sugar reading was almost 700. And with your background as an RN you already know that diabetes is a disease that you must learn to live with. We don't cure it. Once you have it, that's it. You just do what you have to do. It's really amazing that you are still on your feet with a reading that high."

"But I've been sticking other people. I'm not about to have others stick me. I just don't want to be on that end of the needle."

The doctor laughed. "Oh, you'll get used to it. Needles aren't any good unless they have two ends."

That was September 1946. I was twenty-five years old, and probably had been diabetic for some time before that, but just didn't realize it. I did know that sometimes I was terribly thirsty. I would perspire heavily on occasions without realizing why. But my mind was not open to the possibility that I might be classified as a diabetic.

Since then I've learned that there are thousands who are diabetic and don't know it. Sometimes it seems we all want to postpone bad news as long as possible. But in my case it was not an intentional postponement. I simply hadn't thought about it happening to me.

Now here I was with a husband, a little boy, and expecting to become a mother again in December. What a jolt to find that I had the kind of diabetes in which the blood sugar could not be controlled with oral medication. Daily insulin injections would be necessary.

I had visions of scars if I used my arms as the location of frequent insulin injections, so I decided that I would stick myself in another less visible location. On the first time I chased myself around the room three times before I could make the needle catch up.

CHAPTER 2

LOOKING BACK

I was just about to write that's how it all began, but then I realized that one can't really tell a life story beginning at age twenty five. It began way back in 1921, on January 11, in the Lutheran hospital in Des Moines, Iowa, my first day on earth. Ironically that was the year Dr. Banting and his associates in Canada discovered insulin in the pancreas of a fetal calf, leading to its later production from the pancreas of pigs. It's almost as if the good Lord was planning ahead, providing in advance for a little girl who weighed in at two pounds, two ounces, and would some day need insulin.

Of course I can't remember, but I have been told that no one expected me to live. They put me in a shoe box, and Aunt Bell sat up all night knitting a little dress for my burial. The Catholic priest brought ministry, and I was also blessed or christened in a couple of other churches. But I fooled everybody. I survived. This was not the common occurrence those days. The care of low birth weight babies was not nearly so well understood nor technically supported as it is now.

In her first marriage my mother had two girls, Rita and Jane, who I came to know as my older sisters. In her second marriage there were two boys,

Joe and Jack Brown. Then I
came along.

I never knew my father because he died in Excelsior
Springs, in October 1920, a few
months before I was born. He
was from England and made his
living as a church organist.
When he became ill he went to
Excelsior Springs to take advan-
tage of the supposedly health-
giving mineral waters. He played
for churches while he was trying
to regain his health. When he
died it was said that he had
Brights Disease. I have won
dered since if it was not really
diabetes which is inherited.

My mother was a widow with
four children, me on the way,
and needing to somehow make
a living. In Boone, Iowa, not a
long way from Des Moines, lived

my mother's Aunt Mayme, and her husband Clement Malcor. They had no children but had supplied a home to several children who had need of help. Shortly after my birth they came to Des Moines and offered to take me so my mother could get a job and take care of the other four.

So my very early years were in Boone. About the time my elementary school experience began we moved to Aurora, Illinois, where my "dad," whom everyone called "Pop Malcor," was employed as school custodian.

After high school, the Malcors made it possible for me to attend Graceland College in Lamoni, Iowa, where I was known on campus as Betsy Malcor. There I met my future husband, but didn't know it. I didn't have any expectation of seeing him again after leaving campus in the spring of 1939. We had never dated. He was just someone I knew and remembered mainly because my roommate married his brother. I went on to Northwestern University School of Nursing in Evanston, Illinois, and received my RN in February 1942.

By the autumn of 1942 I was part of the VNA, the shorthand way of saying, Visiting Nurses Association, and doing home health work. By this time Wayne had completed his work at the University of Wisconsin and was a minister. We met again in June of 1943 in Aurora where he was holding a series of meetings. I have always remembered the moment when I saw him and he recognized me in the congregation. I decided right then that I would marry him.

In October 1944 I did. A longtime friend from Australia, Walter Johnson, was the minister. It was in a church at 2917 Tracy in Kansas City, beautifully decorated by a little English custodian named Fred Furness who loved flowers and also thought highly of the groom and his bride. And we loved and appreciated him. A few years later we helped raise money to send him on a long overdue trip to his homeland.

After our meeting in Aurora and until we were married we exchanged many letters. Mine were always signed "Mary." So in the years since, I have been

Mary or Mary Elizabeth to those who know me depending on at what point along the way we became acquainted. Only a few friends of my early life still call me Betsy. One of these was a good friend of Aunt Mayme. She was 104 on June 1, 1999. We attended her birthday party and it was she who said early in the gathering, "When do we eat?"

All this had been happening and life had been moving along in rather ordinary although interesting ways. And now this! I just couldn't accept being a diabetic as if it were just another routine assignment. But in the end the doctor convinced me. I had no other choice.

Dr. Link had been our doctor for all the time we had been in

Kansas City, and had become not just our doctor, but a really comfortable and trusted friend. He convinced me there was no other course of action that made sense. I simply must adjust my thinking to accommodate being needled for the rest of my life.

The key was to think of it as another routine procedure which I must build into my daily habits. I set out to do just that. I would carefully avoid thinking of myself as an invalid, and would continue to fulfill my role as a mother and homemaker as well as I could and consider being diabetic as just another personal characteristic like having freckles, disliking garlic, or being afraid of snakes. The needle work would have to become as routine as washing my face or brushing my hair.

CHAPTER 3

SEPTMBER AGAIN

It was a long way to December. I kept getting bigger and bigger. With extreme care and kindness, Dr. Link told me I probably should not expect a live baby. But I fooled them again. On December 19th we became the parents of an eleven pound baby girl with thick curly black hair, dimples, and a mind of her own. Our little boy had a baby sister. And the next day my blood sugar was normal. No more needles!

What a relief! I had gotten used to sticking my finger with a lancet to draw a little blood to test for sugar content. But I didn't like it. And then following that with an insulin needle. I refused to allow myself to think about it anymore than necessary. But even so, it was a wonderful bit of news that my blood sugar was normal within a day or two after the birth of our daughter.

For a while life looked pretty good. But apparently the doctors thought something strange was going on. My experience was not running true to the usual expectations of the medical wise men. September came again and during a visit to the doctor's office for a routine check-up, another doctor asked me to take a glucose tolerance test.

I was asked to drink as much as I could from a pitcher of

sugar-loaded orange juice, and my blood sugar readings were taken at certain time intervals after that to determine how well my body was handling the sugar. Looking back now I recognize that was a normal and appropriate procedure, and even at this time it is still a common practice.

I failed the test in spectacular fashion. Very soon I was in a diabetic coma from which there was considerable doubt about my survival. Dr. Link sat with me all night, and sometime the next day I began to come around. He told me later that he hadn't had very high expectations for me during the long hours of his watch. But I fooled them again.

Now I was back on insulin. For a while it was only twice each day. A lancet to test, and a needle to inject the insulin. Then it became three times a day. Oh, did my fingers get sore!

This has been going on all these years. I was so thankful Dr. Banting was so dedicated to finding answers to questions about diabetes before 1920, and that so many others have found better ways of doing the things I need to do to continue for so long even though I was just outside heaven's front door so often.

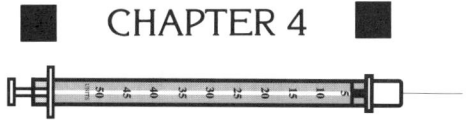

CHAPTER 4

ANOTHER DOCTOR AND VALUABLE FRIEND

During the next fifty plus years there were many more memorable ways in which circumstances had crucial impact on my journey with diabetes. In 1950 we moved to Detroit. We had heard from many sources about the Drs. Shute in London, Ontario, which was not too far from our new home.

On our early visits to the Shute Institute we became aware that the Drs. Shute, Evan, Wilfrid, and Wallace, were checking and testing the use of Vitamin E for various medical problems involving its use as an antioxidant and exploring its value in improving circulation. We became acquainted with considerable numbers of their patients and heard their stories. They had established impressive results.

The Drs. Shute were also highly respected by some people who raised and raced horses in Canada. Of course, I can't remember any statistics, and didn't care much about their interest in the performance of horses. But their reports were impressive. Dr. Evan Shute also prescribed Vitamin E for both my husband and me, telling us that we would do well to continue taking it for the rest of our lives.

While in Detroit we also became acquainted with and found a friend in Carl Muir who was in the business of selling Vitamin E and other medications. He had confidence in Dr. Shute and was careful to make sure we did not fall prey to some who were selling products labeled Vitamin E, but didn't have the same content. He said many people were misled or uninformed and that even among many doctors, Vitamin E was unappreciated and avoided.

Dr. Evan Shute didn't want to become involved in marketing a product that would make it appear that he had a financial rather than a purely scientific motivation in his research and exploration. He had referred us to Mr. Muir and his company who taught us to avoid a syn-

thetic form of the medication
by being sure that the label
said d-alpha and not dl-alpha.
All these years we have fol-
lowed his advice. We were
feeling secure that we had
been well informed on that
particular aspect of our health
care, when at the end of four
years we returned to Independence.

It has been amazing how
many people have had sugges-
tions as to what I should do.
Dozens of people over the
years have told me about
someone who supposedly had
tremendous success overcom-
ing diabetes by the use of
some potion or procedure. Everyone I met was so very so-
licitous about my welfare.
Some ridiculed the use of Vita-

min E. I soon learned as kindly and pleasantly as possible to thank them for the information, but also realized that to try every solution suggested would be very dangerous. I learned the meaning and limitations of "anecdotal evidence."

One of the most recent of these experiences occurred when a longtime friend who much more recently than I had become a diabetic, enthusiastically recommended that I begin using Rezulin, a new product that was just being placed on the market. He seemed so delighted that it was working so well for him. Surely I should try it. I thanked him, of course, but made no commitment or change in the regimen that I had been following.

It was not a bit surprising to me when a few weeks later this same good friend told me he had found it necessary to discontinue the use of that wonderful new product.

"I found out it isn't working for me. I had to quit or it would have killed me." I have since learned that some patients are doing very well with Rezulin, but only if their liver function is checked regularly.

I know, of course, that such experiences do little to establish any conclusions about the many panaceas suggested from time to time. But there seems to be a pattern there because of so many similar instances in the past. Long experience has taught me the value of sticking (!) with established medical procedures and to be very careful about making changes to unproven medications.

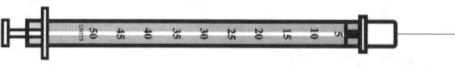

CHAPTER 5

FORTUNATE MOVES

It was in August of 1954 when we moved back to Independence. The temperature was reported to be 114 degrees. The car had no air conditioning. Friends had given us a small aquarium and two goldfish as a parting gift. But even though whenever we stopped along the way our two kids kept the aquarium moving to keep more oxygen in the water, the goldfish didn't make it.

By this time we were awakening to the idea that we should be buying a house instead of renting, so the next year we found a little Andes and Roberts house in Westwood Hills and with a timely gift from Clement Malcor added to our own minuscule savings we were able to make a down payment.

We were now in a neighborhood where there were lots of little children, and we soon noticed that we seemed to be much less than 50% of our childrens' social environment. They were spending most of their playtime outside the house and learning new and colorful words we had not taught them. They were making it necessary for me to check too often to see where they were and what they were doing.

One day we saw a for sale sign on another little house, older, and obviously a long time fixture on a two acre lot with some nice trees. So in less than a year we sold, bought, and moved again.

Our years in the home on T.C. Lea Road were hard work for me, but I enjoyed them as much as I could with my skin being punctured six times a day, three for testing and three for insulin. Dr. Link was again our doctor, and he guided me as I continued to try treating my diabetes as a normal aspect of life. It never got to be fun, but there were many good days and I look back on our time in that old house with pleasant memories. We often laugh as we recall the time we saw two mother cats carrying the same kitten to a new secret hideout. We still have a picture of that scene.

When 1960 came we were asked to take an assignment in London, Ontario. What a move that was going to be! In the previous week our beautiful Collie dog had presented us with thirteen squirming, lovely pups. We also had some sheep and two Hereford calves. Our daughter had a horse, and there were a number of cats to be concerned about. And, oh yes,there was the goat. He had been given to me one time while Wayne was away on a trip. I remember he hadn't seemed very enthusiastic when he came home and found that our menagerie had grown by one little fellow named Smoky. Wayne seemed to have a more vivid mental picture of the growth rate of goats than I did.

We were in town, but the place had been outside the city when we bought it so our animals were legal under a "grandfather" stipulation in the zoning laws. Also, across the street we had acquired a barn and some more land which made the situation tolerable. But Smoky stayed on our side of the street and was always fully aware when I went to the backyard. I often had to race him to the door.

Among our favorite memories is the way we disposed of all those animals in preparation for our move, and without missing a beat in the needle routine. We certainly couldn't take them to Canada. We had no aspirations to be like Abraham going along with his flocks and herds when we came to the Canadian border.

We tried to give the pups away by advertising them as free, with little success. Then we advertised them for $3 each and could have sold a dozen more. We left our daughter's horse on a nearby farm with a friend who had a little girl who thought it was a great idea. The sheep were readily sold and the cats were placed in good homes. Wayne talked to a farmer friend who thought his neighbor might want Smoky and asked him to check it out to be sure, and if so to please come by and get the goat anytime. One day we came home to find pinned to the screen door an unsigned note that read simply "I got your goat."

Now what does all this have to do with my story about being a diabetic? Two points stand out for me in retrospect. First, it shows that, although life is complicated and rather hectic, one can live with diabetes, even the very brittle kind. I'm sure it helped for me to be busy and have lots of things to think about in addition to all those needle pricks.

The other important aspect of that move was that it took us to London, where we again were patients of Dr. Evan Shute. I'm sure that happening was a big influence in keeping me alive so long. Our stay there was only for two and a half years, but during that time I was reinforced in my decision to keep taking the prescribed amount of Vitamin E.

Also it was a time in which I was able to reduce my daily activity to a more reasonable load as compared with the previous six years on those acres in Independence. But in London there was always plenty to do to keep me active.

I could say, as many others would in a similar situation, that the Lord was looking after me. But wasn't He always? I have trouble thinking about God being there and reaching out to save someone in a car accident when someone else in the same car was killed. I find it difficult to believe He specifically makes those selections. I can't believe He loves one of us more than another.

I find it easier to think He is always there for all of us, and that we can depend on His care both here and hereafter. So that the determination of what happens to whom is usually made by us on a cause and effect basis in the natural order of things, although He undoubtedly intervenes in special ways whenever He wants to. It surely seems that He did for me. But we are responsible for our own actions. If we make a mistake, or are killed he still loves us. We just are then in a different place. He can love us anywhere.

While we were in London one of my medical concerns was my eyes. Of course I had become aware that diabetics are always under threat of losing their sight. They often have circulatory problems as well. Amputations and heart problems are common companions of diabetes. I knew that I must give attention to preventing such catastrophes. And I also knew that it was of extreme importance for me to keep my weight under control.

One day I made an appointment with an ophthalmologist. When he learned my medical history and checked my eyes he said, "You are defying statistics. Ninety eight percent of diabetics who have been diabetic for twenty years are blind."

I don't believe the figures are that bad today, because of progress in medical knowledge, and I had no way of knowing if he was right, even then. But I never forgot what he said. Imagine my thoughts when several years later, in Denver, another ophthalmologist said almost the same words to me. I knew I was doing something right. Maybe two things! Even three!

I was staying thin, rarely going over about 120 pounds.

I was trying to keep my needle sticking as regular as possible, in order to remove time as one of the variables. And I was taking Vitamin E daily.

Maybe I should just make it simple and say that the Lord was taking care of me, and I know He was. But I like to think that He was doing so by utilizing my own will as an instrument for my own good. I had heard a story about an old man who was always saying things to children about how the Lord takes care of him. One of his listeners said, "God must love you very much."

The old man responded with a merry twinkle and ascending inflection, "Oooooh yeeesss! I'm one of his favorites." Then after a brief pause he added in an ordinary tone, "Everybody is."

It was that feeling of being one of God's children that helped me through many rough moments. But I never allowed myself to believe that He wanted to do the job alone. He always wanted me to be in the program too. And my husband and I and many well wishers often made sure that my problem was in-cluded in prayers which I am sure He was pleased to hear.

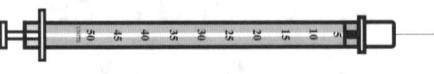

CHAPTER 6

STILL LEARNING

We left London on December 11, 1962 to return again to Independence. It was a very blizzardy day all across the state of Michigan, and I kept hoping that the truck carrying our badly-worn furniture would get lost and I could get new things for our old home. But that was not to be. We arrived safe and sound, furniture still intact but even more worn and scratched, both kids in high school, no animals to take care of, and still six needle pricks every day. Life goes on.

Soon I was at work as a

school nurse in the Independence schools, helping with all kinds of health matters, including vaccinations, and even encouraging some children who needed help in adjusting to the regimen of diabetes. The son of one of my best friends was a little boy who had the task of testing and needling every day just as I did. He has grown to be a fine man who has worked many years for TWA. His son is not a diabetic. He is a college graduate and a promising young opera singer in New York.

The job of school nurse required a car. A friend allowed me, for a time, to use an old and long convertible, for which I was grateful. But I felt terribly conspicuous whenever I drove into the school parking lots. Sometimes it would not start until I lifted the hood and pounded on a thing the owner told me was a solenoid, whatever that is. But it worked.

Soon we bought a well-used 1963 Chevrolet that I drove for a while, then exchanged for a little Triumph which I called Tweety Bird. I loved that little car but the time came when repairs were needed. The repair company also sold cars and suggested we might want to trade for something new. He showed us a little red Toyota sedan, a type that was just being introduced to the Kansas City market. We had never heard of that kind of car, and believed the salesman who said it was from one of the first boatloads from Japan. Best of all, he offered $1,400 for the Triumph, and asked $2,000 for the new Toyota. We added $250 to install air conditioning, and I was in car heaven.

At the end of four years we moved again, this time to Denver where we spent eight wonderful years. We liked the climate; we liked the people. We lived in one nice house for a while, but then had another one built on the southeast part of town where we had a wonderful view of the mountains.

I had become quite weary in school nursing, and when we moved to Denver I quit working but kept the little red sedan. Later when we moved to Washington we sold it because I was uncertain about wanting to drive in the traffic of the east. In the following years we spent time in Washington, D.C., and Des Moines, and then back to the KC area again. This time it was at Lake Tapawingo in Blue Springs, with both kids married, three wonderfully sharp and good looking grandsons, some new furniture mixed with the old, and still six skin pricks every day, rain or shine.

On March 4, 1992 I was in the office of Dr. William Quick, a diabetic specialist who had suggested that my target blood sugar should be 160 which although high for normal, was a reasonable goal for me. He also had urged that I not exceed 120 pounds in weight and complimented me each time I checked in at around 115.

On that day he listened to my heart, and asked if I would mind having a doctor from the office of my primary physician, Dr. Lee Pickering, check me, too. We went down the hall to another office where my heart rate was checked again. Then together they told me the startling news. I should go immediately to the hospital in a wheel chair. I should not even return home.

The next day I had a heart attack and in the next few days had two more, and also a stroke. Most of this time I didn't know much of what was going on. There were three code blues, an angiogram and an angioplasty, and two strokes. My husband and our two kids, then in their forties, have supplied me with most of what I know of the time in the hospital. The highlight memory for them was the kindly way in which one of the cardiologists drew them aside and tried to prepare them for my demise.

Wayne says he distinctly remembers the phrase, "Might not survive this episode" while almost at the same moment another doctor in my room in intensive care was saying, "Oh, I'm getting a pulse." So I fooled them again.

And do you know what? For a little while I was not on six needle sticks a day. They were comparatively few, but they were a lot bigger. The IV in my arm relieved me for a little while from my daily testing and sticking duties.

Now it's a little more than seven years later. I'm still performing the daily rituals. In January of this year I had another heart catheterization and the doctors told me that the large arteries of my heart cannot be opened again. They also say that heart surgery is not possible with my diabetic heart. I must just keep on with my medications, make do with the amount of blood that the small arteries can supply, and keep on with the six skin punctures a day.

In the morning I take two kinds of insulin, humolog and NPH. Wayne pulls them for me and combines them in one needle. The other two times a day I sometimes load the needle myself, and I always stick myself. The other medications are a bunch of pills which Wayne counts out for me.

I'm happy that thousands of diabetics can handle the problem with oral medications. And I'm thankful that day after day I'm fooling folks again even though I require insulin. I hope I can keep it up for a long time.

CHAPTER 7

THE FORWARD LOOK

It is reassuring to note there is considerable effort being made every year to discover more about diabetes and how to control or eradicate it. Every year it seems that some other great breakthrough is just around the corner. Once you begin looking at the news through the eyes of a long-term diabetic you keep noticing how many great discoveries are announced and then later found to be inadequate or dangerous because of side effects and are never heard of again.

The American Diabetes Association keeps looking for a cure by promoting research in various laboratories. I don't know how many years I have belonged but their magazine, *Diabetes Forecast*, continues to give encouragement and report the efforts of researchers. It is wonderful that some diabetics can use an insulin pump to avoid the needle work. Many are able to use only oral medications. The latest product I have heard about is the recently approved Avandia which seems to hold promise for diabetics who are not required to take insulin. It is said to prevent loss of eyes and feet and to delay the need for insulin.

Time will tell how it works out.

Two recent events have helped my morale. I just renewed my Missouri driver's license, which will now expire March 3, 2004. It took some nerve for me to apply because of my age and the possibility that my eyes may have deteriorated.

For the past three or four years I haven't been driving, but having the license has helped me continue with the attitude that diabetes is just a condition of life to be accepted and dealt with just as any other personal circumstance. In addition, passing the examination, including the vision test, was psychological reinforcement for me. We have the prettiest car we ever owned, a ten-year-old Buick LeSabre, and I know I can drive it legally anytime an occasion requires it. Wayne says it is burgundy because he knew I didn't want another red one!

The second recent event, which would be almost meaningless to anyone else but which is gratifying to a long-term diabetic is my receiving a citation and a medal from the Eli Lilly Company for using their product, insulin, for so long. Our son heard about their program and suggested they might want to check my story. It was a surprise to me to receive the recognition. I should be giving **them** an award for producing a medication that was so vital to my survival.

One day not long ago Wayne calculated the number

of times I have punctured my skin as more than 115,000 times. He excluded an estimate of the number of times when using the lancet to get blood for testing I hit a "dry well" and would have to try again. Using a new lancet doesn't seem to help much, but I do carefully use a new needle each time for the insulin.

Because I was able to treat the testing and needling as a routine matter, my long-term dependency on insulin hasn't unduly reduced my activity. I just kept going. I've seen most of the east coast from Campobello at the tip of Maine to Washington, D.C. I also saw Orlando and Disney World.

I rode one day along Bourbon Street in New Orleans. The

San Diego Zoo was enjoyable.
San Francisco and the bridge
were interesting and still are
special because the American
Field Service student from
India who lived with us when
our daughter was a high school
senior now lives near the
north end of the bridge.

I stood on the deck of the
USS Missouri while it was
docked at Bremerton, and
saw the place where General
MacArthur signed the papers
ending World War II. I recently
noted with interest that the
ship is now berthed in Hawaii.
And this brings back memories
of standing on the beautiful
memorial in Pearl Harbor and
looking down at the sunken
Arizona.

We saw the tall tower in

Seattle when it was being completed. In Canada we saw Vancouver, Banff, and Lake Louise. We saw Edmonton, Calgary, and Winnipeg. On one occasion we drove along the St. Lawrence River and visited Montreal and Quebec. At Toronto we saw one of the three World Fairs I have visited. It was interesting to see the ships lifted up at Sault Ste. Marie. Manitoulin and Mackinac Islands were lovely in summer.

Chicago, Detroit, St. Louis, and Salt Lake City all hold memories for me. From our front porch in Denver we could see Pike's Peak, Mt. Evans, and Longs Peak. We went as high as we were allowed on all three. Near Mexico City we climbed to the very top of a high pyramid.

In October of 1994 we celebrated our 50th anniversary at the Clubhouse in Woodmoor, the housing development where we live in President Truman's hometown. We watched from the steps of another church across the street when he and Mrs. Truman arrived at the church for their daughter's wedding and observed Mrs. Truman's obviously frustrating efforts to move him along as he kept stopping to greet people.

I know that many people among the good friends we find here have problems more serious than mine. But life goes on. I find myself being uncomfortable with feeling that I have been so much more greatly blessed than has been my ability to be of use to others.

But as long as the blessings of the good life continue, I will continue to be thankful for the many opportunities which have been mine. I could make this a much longer book by telling you how great our three grandsons are, but I will deny myself that pleasure.

It is my desire and expectation that someone who is a diabetic will read this and be encouraged to keep going even if the road seems rough at times. I believe everyone whose names I have mentioned in this writing, except my family, Dr. Quick, and Dr. Pickering are gone.

In response to the care and concern so many people have provided me, I am pleased to increase their gift to human well being by arranging that proceeds from this work, if any, will be given to our favorite charity.

I wish I could express my thanks individually to so many who have helped me in so many ways in good times and bad. If when you read this, I have already found myself permanently relieved of all this needling, you can be sure I will be saying my thanks again to the One who made this journey so interesting and kept me here so long and helped me fool so many people so many times.

The End

To My Readers

I hope my abbreviated story has been helpful to you.

If you are a diabetic you may want to keep this book and also have a friend read it.

There are two ways to do this. First, you might lend this one. Or, if you prefer, and especially if you want to share with several friends, you might give them the number 1-800-767-8181 and your friends can obtain their own copy on the basis of your recommendation. Either way, you will be a friend.

MEU

For additional copies call
1-800-767-8181
1-816-373-4065

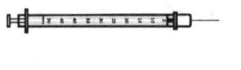